Age-Defying Strength: The 6-Minute Fitness Revolution for 60+

"Reclaim Your Vitality with Simple Exercises At Home Within 21 Days "

By

Dr Sylvia T. Gray

TABLE OF CONTENT

INTRODUCTION

In a world that constantly emphasizes the importance of youth and vitality, aging can sometimes feel like an uphill battle. Yet the truth is that aging is an inevitable part of life. However, it doesn't mean that we have to surrender to its effects. We can choose to age gracefully, maintaining our strength, balance, and energy well into our 60s, 70s, and beyond.

Welcome to "Age-Defying Strength: The 6-Minute Fitness Revolution for 60+," a comprehensive guide that will transform the way you approach fitness and well-being as you age. If you've ever felt like the years have taken a toll on your physical abilities, if you've experienced a decline in energy, or if you're worried about maintaining your independence, this book is your roadmap to a brighter, more vibrant future.

In these pages, you will discover a revolutionary approach to fitness tailored specifically for those in the 60+ age group. We understand the unique challenges and concerns that come with aging, and we've designed a program that empowers you to reclaim your strength, balance, and energy.
The best part? It will only take 6 minutes a day, and in just 21 days, you'll start to experience profound improvements in your well-being.

This book isn't just about exercise; it's about regaining your sense of agency and control over your body. It's about feeling and looking your best, no matter your age. Whether you're an active senior looking to maintain your physical prowess or someone who's been more sedentary but is ready for a positive change, our program is adaptable to your needs.

"Age-Defying Strength" is not a quick-fix solution but a sustainable and practical lifestyle approach. You will learn not just the 'how' but also the 'why' behind each exercise and the science that supports it. We aim to empower you with knowledge so you understand the incredible benefits you'll experience by committing just a few minutes a day to your well-being.

In this book, you will find exercises that you may do at home, at work, or anywhere you have some space and time. You will also find detailed instructions for each exercise, as well as safety tips and common mistakes to avoid. You will learn how to "warm up" and "cool down" effectively and how to "adjust the intensity" and "duration" of your workouts according to your fitness level and goals. You will also find sample workout plans for different conditions, such as when you are traveling, recovering from an injury, or when you want to challenge yourself.

This book is not only based on the latest scientific research but also on the real-life experiences of people who have successfully followed the 6-minute fitness approach. You will read inspiring stories and testimonials from people who have improved their bodies and lives with this simple and effective method. You will also find solutions to frequently asked questions, myths, and misconceptions about strength training and aging. You will also get access to a supportive network of fellow 6-minute fitness fanatics, where you can share your progress, ask questions, and get feedback.

Age-Defying Strength, The 6-Minute Fitness Revolution for 60+ is not just a book. It is a lifestyle shift that will help you live longer, healthier, and happier. It is a present that you may give yourself and your loved ones. It is a challenge that you can take on and overcome. It is a revolution that you can join and lead. So, are you ready to defy age and become stronger than ever? If you're ready to embark on a transformative journey, if you're eager to take control of your aging process and emerge stronger, more balanced, and bursting with energy, let's begin because your best years are ahead of you, and they start right here, in these pages; therefore, acquire your copy of this book today and start your 6-minute fitness journey!

CHAPTER 1

Embracing Your 60s and Beyond

In ments in healthcare, a heightened focus on holistic well-being, and a collective desire for an active and fulfilling life, the landscape of aging is undergoing a profound transformation. While aging naturally brings physical changes and unique challenges, it's crucial to recognize that it doesn't have to equate to a decline in your quality of life. Your 60s and beyond can be a time of significant personal growth and enjoyment if approached with the right mindset.

Wellness is a central focus of the new mindset on aging. People are increasingly realizing that maintaining physical and mental health is not just for the young but is equally important as we age. With this approach, seniors are encouraged to stay active, engage in lifelong learning, and embrace a balanced and healthy lifestyle. As a result, older adults are more proactive in taking charge of their health by engaging in regular exercise, practicing good nutrition, and paying attention to their mental well-being. The concept of "aging well" is not only attainable but is increasingly becoming a shared aspiration.

Maintaining independence and a high quality of life has become a central goal for seniors. The right mindset fosters the belief that you can live life on your terms, pursue your passions, and remain self-sufficient. This is not just about growing old; it's about growing in wisdom and experience. As a result, seniors should engage in an adventure. travel, engage in new hobbies, and participate in stress-free activities in their communities.

Many are defying traditional retirement age norms and continuing to work, not out of necessity but for personal fulfillment and a sense of purpose. The right mindset places a strong emphasis on lifelong learning. Seniors should embrace opportunities to expand their knowledge and skills. Whether it's pursuing higher education, learning a new language, or taking up a musical instrument, older adults are demonstrating that the quest for knowledge is ageless.

The Power of Mindset in Aging Gracefully

Aging is inevitable, but how we age is largely influenced by our mindset. Our thoughts and beliefs about aging can have a profound impact on our physical and mental health, our happiness, and our longevity. In this article, we will explore how positive thinking can help seniors age gracefully and enjoy their golden years.

What is positive thinking?

Positive thinking is not about ignoring reality or being unrealistic. It is about focusing on the good aspects of life, being optimistic about the future, and having a sense of purpose and meaning. Positive thinking can also involve cultivating gratitude, forgiveness, humor, curiosity, and resilience.

Positive thinking can benefit seniors in many ways, such as

Enhancing physical health: Positive thinking can lower the risk of age-related diseases, such as heart disease, diabetes, and Alzheimer's disease. It can also boost the immune system, reduce inflammation, and promote healing. Positive thinking can also motivate seniors to adopt healthy behaviors, such as exercising regularly, eating well, and staying hydrated.

Improving mental health: Positive thinking can protect seniors from depression, anxiety, and cognitive decline. It can also enhance memory, attention, creativity, and problem-solving skills. Positive thinking can also help seniors cope with stress, adversity, and loss and foster a sense of well-being and satisfaction.

Increasing social connection: Positive thinking can make seniors more attractive, likable, and supportive of others, and thus improve their relationships with family, friends, and the community. It can also help seniors find new opportunities for social engagement, learning, and volunteering, thus expanding their social network and reducing loneliness.

Extending lifespan: Positive thinking can add years to seniors' lives and, more importantly, quality to those years. A 2019 study found that positive thinking can result in an 11–15% longer lifespan and a stronger likelihood of living to age 85 or older.

How can seniors develop positive thinking?

Positive thinking is not a fixed trait that some people have and others don't. It is a skill that can be learned and practiced, regardless of age or circumstances.

Here are some tips for seniors to cultivate positive thinking

Challenge negative thoughts: Negative thoughts are often distorted, exaggerated, or irrational and can lead to negative emotions and behaviors. Seniors can learn to identify and challenge these thoughts and replace them with more realistic, balanced, and positive ones. For example, instead of thinking "I'm too old to learn anything new", seniors can think "I have a lifetime of experience and wisdom to draw from, and I can always learn something new if I try".

Practice gratitude: Gratitude is the appreciation of what's treasured and significant in life. Seniors can practice gratitude by keeping a journal, writing thank-you notes, expressing gratitude to others, or simply reflecting on the good things that happen each day. Gratitude can help seniors focus on the positive aspects of their lives and increase their happiness and optimism.

Forgive and let go: Forgiveness is the act of releasing resentment, anger, or bitterness towards oneself or others who have caused harm or offense. Seniors can practice forgiveness by acknowledging their feelings, empathizing with the other person, and deciding to move on. Forgiveness can help seniors heal from past hurts, reduce stress, and improve their mental and physical health.

Laugh and have fun: Humor is the ability to see the funny or absurd side of life and to laugh at oneself or the situation. Seniors can practice humor by watching comedies, reading jokes, playing games, or spending time with people who make them laugh. Humor can help seniors cope with difficulties, lighten up their mood, and enhance their creativity and social skills.

Be curious and keep learning: Curiosity is the desire to know more about oneself, others, or the world. Seniors can practice curiosity by asking questions, exploring new places, trying new things, or taking up new hobbies. Curiosity can help seniors stimulate their brains, expand their horizons, and discover new sources of joy and meaning.

Be resilient and adaptable: Resilience is the ability to bounce back from challenges, setbacks, or changes. Seniors can practice resilience by accepting reality, focusing on solutions, seeking support, and finding the silver lining. Resilience can help seniors overcome obstacles, grow from adversity, and adjust to new situations.

Positive thinking is a powerful tool for seniors to age gracefully and live their best lives. By adopting a positive mindset, seniors can enhance their physical and mental health, increase their social connection, and extend their lifespan. Positive thinking is not a fixed trait but a skill that can be learned and practiced.

Seniors can cultivate positive thinking by challenging negative thoughts, practicing gratitude, forgiving and letting go, laughing and having fun, being curious and keeping learning, and being resilient and adaptable. By doing so, seniors can not only age well but also age happily.

Common concerns and misconceptions about exercise for seniors

A lot of seniors are hesitant to begin or maintain an exercise regimen because of typical misunderstandings and worries. We will dispel some of these beliefs and provide you with the facts about physical activity for older adults.

Myth: Exercise will not improve the physical frailty and weakness of older individuals.

Fact: Regardless of your age or level of fitness right now, exercise can really help you get stronger, more resilient, and more mobile. Numerous chronic conditions that might impair your independence and health, such as diabetes, heart disease, and osteoporosis, can be avoided or delayed with exercise. You can recover from diseases, surgeries, and injuries more quickly if you exercise.

Myth: As we age, our bodies don't require as much physical activity.

Fact: It's the other way around. Your body changes significantly as you age, which may have an impact on your bone density, muscle mass, metabolism, and joint performance. You may be more vulnerable to weight gain, balance issues, and decreased mobility as a result of these changes. You must continue to be active and push your body through regular exercise to counteract these effects. It is recommended by the World Health Organization that people 65 years of age and older engage in muscle-strengthening activities at least twice a week.

Myth: Older individuals who exercise run the risk of hurting themselves. **Fact:** As long as seniors adhere to a few simple rules, most of them can safely and healthily engage in physical activity. You should speak with your doctor and have a medical examination to determine your current state of health and level of fitness before beginning any workout regimen. Additionally, you should steer clear of activities that lead to pain, discomfort, or extreme weariness and instead select workouts that are suitable for your talents and limitations.

Myth: Exercise that is only intense and prolonged is beneficial.

Fact: As long as you engage in regular, enjoyable physical activity, any quantity or kind of exercise can improve your health and well-being. To benefit from exercise, you don't need to run a marathon, lift big weights, or join a gym. There are lots of ways to include exercise into your everyday schedule, such as dancing, walking, gardening, or playing with your grandkids. Finding and sticking to something that fits your preferences, objectives, and lifestyle is crucial.

Exercise benefits your mind and spirit in addition to your physical health. Exercise helps lessen stress, anxiety, and sadness while also improving mood, memory, and cognitive performance. You can feel younger and happier and gain a sense of purpose, accomplishment, and satisfaction from exercising. Don't let rumors and false beliefs prevent you from working out. One of the nicest things you can do for your loved ones and yourself is exercise. Take up fitness now and reap its benefits well into your 60s and beyond.

Enjoy a hassle-free 60s and beyond

Age is simply a number; it doesn't define who you are or what you are capable of. Try not to stress over the figure. Choose to concentrate on the events, memories, accomplishments, and objectives that give your life purpose and fulfillment rather than fretting about the passing of time. Enjoy your successes, but don't let them define who you are.

Learning, growing, and doing new things are never too old for you.

Look after your health, As you age, it's critical to preserve your health, as it's your greatest asset. Consume a diet high in whole grains, fruits, vegetables, lean protein, and healthy fats. Make sure your diet is balanced. Eat less processed food, sugary additions, and salt. Keep your alcohol consumption to a minimum and drink lots of water. Take care of your stress levels and get enough sleep. Work out regularly, incorporating several types of exercises like aerobics, strength, flexibility, and balance training. Make sure to take good care of yourself by scheduling routine exams, screenings, and immunizations. As directed by your physician, take your prescription drugs if you have any long-term health issues.

Continue having sex since it improves both your physical and emotional well-being in addition to being a source of enjoyment. Enhancement of mood, immune system strength, blood pressure lowering, pain reduction, and cardiovascular health are all possible with sex. Through the stimulation of blood flow and the maintenance of toned vaginal muscles, sex can also help you maintain the health of your vagina, particularly after menopause. Aside from enhancing closeness and happiness, sex can fortify your emotional connection to your spouse. Speak with your therapist or physician if you are experiencing problems with desire or sexual function. Enjoying your sexual life at any age is possible with a variety of treatments and remedies.

Live life to the fullest, The 1960s are a fantastic time to follow your passions and fulfill your hobbies and aspirations. You have the time and energy to pursue your passions, whether they be writing, drawing, gardening, traveling, volunteering, or picking up a new skill. Taking up your passions can change your life, increase brain activity, boost your confidence, and introduce you to like-minded individuals. Try new things, and don't be scared to push yourself to get out of your comfort zone. You may pick up new skills or find satisfying pursuits.

Keep in touch, As you get older, social interactions become even more important for your overall health. You may avoid loneliness and isolation, stave off cognitive decline and dementia, and maintain your mental and emotional well-being by maintaining a robust social network. Permit yourself to maintain regular communication with your loved ones and friends. Make friends with people who share your interests, values, or beliefs by joining a club, group, or community. Engage in social activities, events, and get-togethers. Become friends with new people that you meet. Act amiable, cordial, and encouraging. It is always possible to find someone who can make a positive impact on your life.

A positive and growth-oriented mindset is a powerful asset in the process of aging gracefully and maintaining one's quality of life. It can significantly impact good physical health and overall happiness. Research has shown that a positive mindset can lead to better physical health outcomes. Seniors with a growth-oriented mindset are more likely to recover from illnesses and surgeries more quickly. Maintaining strength allows you to carry out daily activities independently. This includes tasks like lifting groceries, climbing stairs, and even just getting in and out of chairs or beds with ease. Strength training and balance exercises can significantly reduce the risk of falls, which is a common concern for seniors. This, in turn, lowers the risk of injuries and fractures.

With age-defying strength, you can enjoy a higher quality of life. You have the physical capacity to engage in a wide range of activities, from traveling and playing with grandchildren to pursuing hobbies and interests. Weight-bearing exercises that come with strength training help maintain bone density, reducing the risk of osteoporosis and fractures. A strong heart and a healthy cardiovascular system can be achieved through regular exercise. This reduces the risk of heart disease, high blood pressure, and other cardiovascular issues.

CHAPTER 2

Unlocking the Science of Aging Gracefully

Understanding the wisdom behind aging is the key to unleashing age-defying strength. In this chapter, we will claw into the natural and physiological changes that occur as we grow older. Armed with this knowledge, you will be better equipped to appreciate why exercise and strength training are essential for maintaining vitality in your 60s and beyond.

The biological reality of aging

Aging is a natural and complex process. At the cellular level, it involves a multitude of changes, including

Muscle loss (sarcopenia): One of the most significant age-related changes is the loss of muscle mass. Starting as early as your 30s, muscle mass tends to drop by about 3–8 per decade, making you weaker over time due to a decrease in the production of muscle cells and an increase in the breakdown of muscle tissue. Muscle loss can affect your balance, coordination, mobility, and endurance. It can also increase your risk of falls, injuries, and fractures.

To prevent or slow down muscle loss, you should include physical activity in your daily routine. Aim for a minimum of one hundred and fifty (150) minutes of moderate-depth cardio exercise per week, consisting of walking, cycling, or swimming.

You should also do some strength training exercises at least twice a week, such as lifting weights, using resistance bands, or doing bodyweight exercises. Strength training can help you build and maintain muscle mass, as well as improve your bone density and metabolism.

Bone viscosity reduction: As you age, your bones may become less thick, making them more susceptible to fractures as a result of an increase in the resorption of existing bone cells and a decrease in the creation of new ones. Osteoporosis, a disorder that weakens, brittles, and increases the risk of fractures, can be brought on by bone loss. Although osteoporosis can damage any bone in the body, it most commonly affects the wrists, hips, and spine.

You should get adequate calcium and vitamin D in your diet to stop or minimize bone loss. Strong bones require the mineral calcium to be built and maintained. The hormone vitamin D aids in the body's absorption and utilization of calcium. For persons over 50, the recommended daily intake of calcium is 1,200 mg, while the recommended daily consumption of vitamin D is 800-IU.

Apart from consuming adequate amounts of calcium and vitamin D, you ought to engage in weight-bearing activities like dancing or jogging. Exercises involving weight bearing can help you promote bone growth and stop bone loss. Additionally, since smoking and drinking too much alcohol can harm your bones, you should abstain from these behaviors.

Metabolism retardation: Your metabolism tends to decelerate, which can lead to weight gain. This is incomplete due to a reduction in muscle mass, which plays a vital part in calorie burning.

Reduced Inflexibility: Joints and muscles may become stiffer, leading to decreased inflexibility.

This can cause discomfort and a reduced range of motion.

Decreased Cardiovascular Capacity: The heart and blood vessels may not work as efficiently, reducing your cardiovascular capacity and stamina.

Cognitive Changes: While cognitive aging is largely variable, some individuals may witness a decline in memory and cognitive function as they progress.

Physiological changes that occur as we grow older

Hormonal Changes: Hormonal changes include a drop in coitus hormones(estrogen and testosterone). These changes can impact sexual health and other bodily functions.

Lung function may drop, reducing the capacity for aerobic exercise and occasionally leading to briefness of breath.

Digestive System: The digestive system may decelerate, leading to issues such as constipation and difficulty absorbing certain nutrients.

Vision Changes: Vision may decline due to changes in the lenses of the eyes because the lens, retina, and optic nerve in the eyes are becoming less healthy and functional. Reading, driving, working, and carrying out daily tasks can all be impacted by vision loss. Injuries, accidents, and falls may also become more likely as a result.

Protecting your eyes from damaging ultraviolet (UV) rays from sources including sunshine, tanning beds, and welding can help stop or slow down vision loss. Additionally, you should visit an optometrist or ophthalmologist on a regular basis to have your eyes examined.

This is especially important if you experience any symptoms of vision loss, such as hazy or flashing eyes, difficulty seeing at night, or strange vision. Using glasses, contact lenses, or other corrective equipment that can enhance your vision and quality of life is something you should think about if you suffer from vision loss.

Hearing Changes: Hearing loss may occur, frequently starting with difficulty hearing high-pitched sounds because of a breakdown in the cochlea, auditory nerve, and hair cells—all components that make up the inner ear. Your capacity to interact with others, communicate, and enjoy life can all be impacted by hearing loss. It may also raise your chances of loneliness, depression, and cognitive decline.

Protecting your ears from excessive noise exposure, such as loud music, machinery, or fireworks, can help prevent or slow down hearing loss.

Additionally, you ought to have a professional evaluation of your hearing on a regular basis, particularly if you experience any symptoms of hearing loss, like difficulty understanding conversations, having to ask people to repeat themselves, or turning up the TV or radio volume.

If you have trouble hearing, you should think about using assistive technology hearing aids, such as the invisible hearing aid known as Audien, which is designed to fit inside the ear canal. Starkeys are tinnitus devices that assist in covering up the buzzing or ringing noise that certain people experience. Simple volume control and an on/off switch characterize Phonak's user-friendly hearing aids. Highly effective and reasonably priced hearing aids from Audicus have excellent sound quality and performance.

You can enhance your quality of life and your hearing with any of the above-mentioned devices.

Immune System: The vulnerable system weakens, making the body more susceptible to infections and ailments. Vaccinations may be less effective.

Cognitive Changes: Cognitive changes can include a gradual decline in memory, recycling speed, and administrative function. While cognitive aging varies among individuals, some degree of decline is common.

Skin Changes: The skin becomes thinner, drier, and less elastic. This can lead to wrinkles, age spots, and increased vulnerability to skin injuries.

It's important to note that while these changes are natural, they can be caused by factors such as genetics, life, and overall health. Maintaining a healthy life, including regular exercise, a balanced diet, and regular medical check-ups, can help alleviate some of these age-related changes and promote overall well-being as we grow older.

The Impact of Lifestyle Decisions and Genetics on Seniors Over 60

You might be curious about the extent to which your lifestyle decisions and genetics impact your longevity as you approach senior year. The answer is complex since both variables have a big impact on how you feel about yourself and how likely you are to get sick. You can, however, take certain actions to maximize your genetic potential and develop wholesome behaviors that can postpone or stop the start of age-related illnesses. In this article, we will discuss some of the major facets of genetics and lifestyle decisions for seniors sixty years of age and older.

Genetics: Your Health's Prescription

The sections of DNA known as your genes are what contain the instructions needed to make proteins, which are the fundamental units of your cells and tissues. Numerous physical and biological characteristics, including blood type, metabolism, and eye color, are inherited. Your parents give you your DNA, and you also share some of your genes with your family members. Certain genes are permanent and unchangeable, but lifestyle and environmental influences can affect other genes.

Your genetic makeup can also affect how susceptible you are to specific illnesses, like diabetes, cancer, Alzheimer's disease, and heart disease. These conditions are referred to as multifactorial disorders because they frequently result from a confluence of environmental and genetic elements. For instance, even if you have a gene that raises your risk of type 2 diabetes, you may be able to avoid the illness if you follow healthy eating guidelines, exercise frequently, and maintain a healthy weight. However, even if you don't have a gene that makes you more likely to get heart disease, you could still get it if you smoke, have high blood pressure, and consume a lot of fat in your diet.

Epigenetics is the study of how environmental influences and genetics interact to influence health. The term "epigenetics" describes modifications to your genes' expression or activity that do not affect the DNA sequence. Numerous factors, including nutrition, stress, smoking, pollution, and aging, might contribute to these alterations. For example, various meals have the ability to either activate or deactivate genes related to immunity, metabolism, or inflammation. Certain epigenetic changes can be passed on to your offspring, while others can be reversed by modifying your lifestyle.

Lifestyle Choices: The Power of Your Habits

Your lifestyle choices are the behaviors and habits that you adopt in your daily life, such as what you eat, how much you exercise, how you cope with stress, how much you sleep, and whether you smoke or drink alcohol. Your lifestyle choices can have a profound impact on your health and longevity, as they can affect your body's functions, your mood, your energy levels, and your risk of developing various diseases.

According to the World Health Organization, about 60% of the global burden of chronic diseases and

80% of the deaths from these diseases are attributable to four modifiable lifestyle factors: a bad diet, bodily inactivity, tobacco use, and the damaging use of alcohol. These factors can lead to obesity, high blood pressure, high cholesterol, diabetes, and other conditions that can damage your organs and systems, such as your heart, brain, kidneys, liver, and bones. By contrast, adopting healthy lifestyle habits can prevent or delay the onset of these diseases, improve your quality of life, and extend your lifespan.

Some of the healthy lifestyle choices that can benefit your health and longevity

eating a balanced diet that is rich in fruits, vegetables, whole grains, lean proteins, healthy fats, and fiber and low in added sugars, salt, saturated fats, and trans fats. A healthy diet can provide you with the nutrients, antioxidants, and phytochemicals that your body needs to function properly, fight infections, repair damage, and prevent inflammation. A healthy diet can also help you maintain a healthy weight, lower your blood pressure and cholesterol, regulate your blood sugar, and reduce your risk of various diseases, such as cardiovascular disease, diabetes, cancer, and dementia.

getting regular physical activity that includes aerobic, strength, and flexibility exercises. Physical activity can improve your cardiovascular fitness, muscle strength, bone density, balance, coordination, and mobility. It can also boost your metabolism, immune system, mood, and cognitive function. Physical activity can help you prevent or manage obesity, hypertension, diabetes, osteoporosis, arthritis, depression, and anxiety. The recommended amount of physical activity for adults aged 65 and older is at least 150 minutes of moderate-intensity or 75 minutes of vigorous-intensity aerobic exercise per week and muscle-strengthening sports activities on extra days in step with the week.

Your stress levels and coping with your emotions in healthy ways Stress can have negative effects on your physical and mental health, as it can trigger the release of hormones that can increase your blood pressure, heart rate, blood sugar, and inflammation. Stress can also impair your immune system, digestion, sleep, memory, and mood. Chronic stress can increase your risk of cardiovascular disease, diabetes, depression, anxiety, and other disorders. To manage your stress, you can practice relaxation techniques such as deep breathing, meditation, yoga, or tai chi. You can also seek social support, express your feelings, engage in hobbies, or seek professional help if needed.

Getting enough sleep and following a regular sleep schedule Sleep is essential for your health and well-being, as it allows your body and brain to rest, recover, and regenerate. Sleep can also enhance your immune system, metabolism, memory, learning, and mood. Lack of sleep or poor sleep quality can impair your physical and mental performance, increase your appetite, lower your immunity, and raise your risk of obesity, diabetes, cardiovascular disease, and cognitive decline. The recommended amount of sleep for adults aged 65 and older is seven to eight hours per night! To improve your sleep, you can avoid caffeine, alcohol, and nicotine before bedtime, limit your exposure to light and noise, follow a relaxing bedtime routine, and keep your bedroom comfortable and dark.

Avoiding or quitting smoking and limiting your alcohol intake Smoking and excessive alcohol consumption can harm your health and longevity, as they can damage your cells, tissues, and organs and increase your risk of various diseases, such as cancer, cardiovascular disease, respiratory disease, liver disease, and neurological disorders. Smoking can also accelerate the aging process, as it can reduce the blood flow to your skin, cause wrinkles, and affect your hair and teeth. Alcohol can also interfere with your sleep, mood, cognition, and coordination. If you smoke, you can seek help from your doctor, a counselor, or a support group to quit. If you drink alcohol, you should do so in moderation, which means no more than one drink per day for women and two drinks per day for men.

Your genes and your lifestyle choices are both important factors that influence your health and longevity. While you cannot change your genes, you can optimize their expression and function by adopting healthy lifestyle habits that can prevent or delay the onset of age-related diseases. By eating a balanced diet, getting regular physical activity, managing your stress, getting enough sleep, and avoiding or quitting smoking and limiting your alcohol intake, you can improve your quality of life and live longer and better.

Exercise slows down the aging process

Physical activity has the potential to mitigate the effects of aging on various fronts, including biological, behavioral, and social. Exercise can increase our health span, or the amount of time we spend in good health and disease-free living, in addition to lengthening our longevity. Additionally, it can raise our level of enjoyment, contentment, and well-being. Consequently, one of the greatest and easiest anti-aging strategies we can use is exercise.

Any frequent, moderate physical activity can provide the same benefits as exercise, regardless of age, gender, or skill. Finding a hobby or activity that we enjoy and that meets our needs and objectives is crucial, as is practicing it regularly and securely.

So let's make use of our bodies and minds and employ exercise to slow down the aging process.

CHAPTER 3

The 6-Minute Fitness Approach for Seniors

In chapter, we introduce the core conception of the 6-Minute Fitness Approach, an acclimatized and time-effective authority designed to help seniors reclaim their strength, balance, and energy. We understand that time constraints and physical limitations can be factors for numerous seniors, so we have developed a program that can be seamlessly integrated into your daily routine.

The 6-Minute Fitness Approach

As we age, preserving top-frame power becomes more and more crucial for average fitness and useful independence.

One powerful workout that may assist seniors in enhancing their upper-body energy is changing push-ups. These modified versions of the conventional push-up are, in particular, designed to cater to the wishes and capabilities of seniors, making them a secure and handy option. In this article, we will explore the various aspects of modified pushups for seniors, including their benefits, techniques, and safety considerations.

Core Engagement and Body Alignment

The importance of engaging the core is crucial during modified push-ups, as it provides stability and support to the entire body. Seniors have to be conscious of drawing the navel closer to the backbone, keeping an impartial backbone position, and warding off immoderate arching or rounding of the back.

Maintaining proper body alignment

Proper body alignment is essential for performing modified push-ups safely and effectively. Seniors need to attempt to preserve an immediate line from the top to the heels at some stage in the exercise. This alignment allows the distribution of the weight flippantly and prevents undue pressure at the joints.

The 6-Minute Fitness Approach is based on the idea that small, harmonious sweats can yield significant results. It's a manageable routine that only requires a few twinkles each day, making it accessible and realistic for seniors in all fitness situations. Then, how does it work?

Holistic Approach: The program addresses multiple aspects of well-being, including strength, balance, and cardiovascular fitness. This holistic approach ensures that you are working from all angles of your health.

Practical exercise methods and

Step-by-Step Guide for Performing Modified Push Ups for Seniors

Knee-supported push-up technique: Begin on all fours, with the knees hip-width aside and the arms barely wider than shoulder-width aside.
Lower the higher frame in the direction of the floor by means of bending the elbows at the same time as keeping a direct line from the head to the knees.
Pause briefly, then push back up to the starting position, fully extending the arms without locking the elbows.
Repeat the desired number of times.

Incline push-up technique: Position yourself dealing with an increased surface, along with a bench or countertop, with the arms positioned shoulder-width aside at the surface.

Walk the feet again to create a diagonal line from head to heels, engaging the core and preserving proper body alignment.

Lower the upper body towards the surface by bending the elbows while keeping the core engaged.

Pause briefly, then push back up to the starting position, fully extending the arms without locking the elbows.

Repeat the desired number of times.

Warm-up (2 twinkles): Begin with a light warm-up to prepare your muscles and joints for exercise. You can do this by walking in place or making gentle arm circles. Warming up helps with injuries.

Strength Training (2 Twinkles): Perform strength training exercises to build and save muscle. Then there are some simple yet effective strength exercises for seniors.

Chair Squats: Stand in front of a sturdy chair, sit back into a squat, and return to a standing position.
Sit with your feet hip-width apart.
Stand up from the chair, and then sit back down.
Ensure your knees stay aligned with your feet and don't go past your toes.
Repeat for 10–15 reps.

Wall push-ups: Stand facing a wall with your arms extended at chest height.
Place your hands on the wall. Step back a bit and lean your body into the wall. Bend your elbows to bring your chest toward the wall and also push back.
repeat for 10–15 reps.

Leg raises: Sit in a sturdy chair with your feet flat on the floor. Lift one leg straight out in front of you. Hold for many seconds and also lower it. Alternate legs and perform 10–15 reps on each leg.

Balance and Inflexibility Exercises for Seniors (1 twinkle)

Work on your balance and inflexibility, which are vital for fall prevention and diurnal mobility. Try these exercises.

Heel-to-Toe Walk: Stand with the heel of one foot touching the toes of the other. Take small steps, placing one foot directly in front of the other and walking in a straight line. Hold your arms out to your sides to help with balance.

Standing leg raises: Stand near a sturdy surface (e.g., a countertop or chair for support). Lift one leg straight up in front of you. Hold for many seconds and also lower it. Switch to the other leg and repeat. Aim for 10–15 leg raises on each leg.

Common Mistakes to Avoid

Collapsed or rounded shoulders: Seniors need to be aware of retaining their shoulders engaged and heading off, disintegrating, or rounding all through the modified push-ups. This helps maintain proper form and prevents unnecessary strain on the shoulders and neck.

Sagging hips or lower back: Seniors need to try to maintain their hips in step with their shoulders and keep away from sagging or overarching the lower back. Proper alignment of the hips and core engagement ensures that the exercise targets the intended muscle groups effectively.

Elbows flaring out: To save you pressure at the shoulders and preserve premiere muscle engagement, seniors ought to aim to hold their elbows pointing barely backward, as opposed to flaring out to the sides, at some stage in the push-up motion.

Cardiovascular Fitness Exercise for Seniors

Marching in Place: Stand with your base hip-range piecemeal. March in place by lifting your knees as high as you can comfortably. Swing your arms in collaboration with your legs. March for one nanosecond to elevate your heart rate and ameliorate cardiovascular health.

Cool Down and Stretching for Seniors After completing your exercises, it's pivotal to cool down and stretch to maintain inflexibility and help with muscle soreness and stiffness. It can also gently and securely lower your blood pressure and heart rate. You can do some light aerobics to help calm down, and there are some essential stretches to follow.

Seated Hamstring Stretch: Sit on the edge of a chair with one leg extended straight. Gently spare forward, keeping your reverse straight, and reach for your toes. Hold for 15–30 seconds on each leg.

Standing quadriceps stretch: Stand next to a sturdy surface for balance. Bend your knee and bring your heel toward your buttocks. Hold your ankle with your hand and gently pull your heel closer to your buttocks. Hold for 15–30 seconds on each leg.

Calf Stretch: Stand near a wall for support. Step one foot back and press your heel into the floor. Keep your aft leg straight and feel the stretch in your calf. Hold for 15–30 seconds on each leg.

Shoulder Stretch: Extend one arm across your chest. Use your other arm to gently pull your extended arm closer to your chest. Hold for 15–30 seconds on each arm.

Do not forget to breathe deeply and relax into each stretch, never forcing your body into uncomfortable positions. Stretching helps maintain and ameliorate your range of motion and inflexibility, reducing the threat of injury.

Benefits of Modified Push-Ups for Seniors

Strengthening the chest, arms, and shoulders Modified push-ups aim at the muscular tissues of the chest, arms, and shoulders, assisting seniors in constructing energy and enhancing muscle tone in those areas. This can enhance typical upper-body functionality and aid normal tasks.

Enhancing core stability and balance: Engaging the core throughout modified push-ups enables seniors to enhance core stability and balance. A strong and stable core is essential for maintaining proper posture, preventing falls, and supporting daily movements.

Improving overall functional strength: By targeting multiple muscle groups in the upper body, modified push-ups contribute to improved overall functional strength. Seniors can revel in expanded ease in performing each daily activity, including lifting, carrying, and pushing.

Tips for Overcoming Challenges

Building upper-body strength gradually: Seniors should start with modified push-ups that suit their current strength level and gradually progress to more challenging variations. Consistency and gradual progression are key to constructing upper-body strength safely and effectively.

Using a chair or support if needed: Seniors who struggle with preserving the right shape or require extra guidance can use a chair or a different stable surface to carry out modified push-ups. This offers greater help while permitting seniors to continue working on their energy and technique.

To maximize the benefits of strength training for your mental health, you should follow some tips and recommendations, such as:

Choose exercises that challenge your brain as well as your muscles, such as complex movements, coordination, balance, and reaction time. Perform strength training in the morning or afternoon, rather than in the evening, to avoid interfering with your sleep quality and quantity.

Combine strength training with aerobic exercise, such as walking, cycling, or swimming, to boost your cardiovascular health and brain function.

Listen to music, podcasts, audiobooks, or other stimulating audio while you strength train to enhance your mood and motivation.
Seek social support and interaction from your strength training partners, instructors, or online communities to increase your enjoyment and adherence.

Listen to your body and take breaks when necessary

It is important for seniors to pay attention to their bodies and take breaks as needed at some stage in their push-up practice. Pushing too hard or ignoring signs of fatigue or pain can boost the chances of injury. Seniors have to honor their personal limits and regulate their workout routines accordingly.

The 6-Minute Fitness Approach is adaptable to your requirements and can be acclimatized to your fitness position. By incorporating these practical exercises into your diurnal routine, you will witness advancements in strength, balance, and inflexibility, contributing to your overall well-being and enhancing your age-defying strength.

Setting realistic goals and expectations for seniors

Setting realistic goals and expectations for seniors is a way of helping them live fulfilling and meaningful lives. Goals can provide motivation, purpose, and direction for older adults, as well as a sense of achievement and satisfaction. However, not all goals are suitable or realistic for seniors, depending on their abilities, limitations, and preferences.

Therefore, it is important to consider some factors when setting goals and expectations for seniors, such as:

The relevance and value of the goal for the senior: The goal should be something that the senior is interested in, passionate about, or wants to learn or improve. It should also align with their values, beliefs, and personal identity. For example, a senior who loves animals may want to volunteer at an animal shelter, while a senior who enjoys reading may want to join a book club.

The difficulty and feasibility of the goal for the senior: The goal should be challenging enough to stimulate the senior's mind and body, but not so difficult that it causes frustration, stress, or disappointment. It should also be feasible within the senior's physical, mental, and financial capabilities, as well as the available resources and support. For example, a senior who has mobility issues may not be able to walk five miles a day, but they may be able to walk for 10 minutes, three times a week, with the help of a walker or a caregiver.

The specificity and measurability of the goal for the senior: The goal should be clear and specific, so that the senior knows exactly what they want to achieve and how to achieve it. It should also be measurable so that the senior can track their progress and evaluate their outcomes. For example, a senior who wants to improve their memory may set a goal to do a crossword puzzle or a Sudoku puzzle every day and record their completion time and accuracy.

The flexibility and adaptability of the goal for the senior: The goal should be flexible and adaptable, so that the senior can adjust it according to their changing needs, preferences, and circumstances.

The goal should not be rigid or fixed, but rather a guide that can be modified or revised as needed. For example, a senior who wants to try out a new restaurant every month may change their plan if they have dietary restrictions, budget constraints, or health issues. By setting realistic goals and expectations for seniors, caregivers can help them achieve a sense of well-being, happiness, and fulfillment.

Caregivers can also support seniors in their goal-setting process by

Managing expectations with realistic goals: caregivers can help seniors set goals that are appropriate for their abilities and limitations and avoid setting goals that are too high or too low. Caregivers can also help seniors understand the benefits and challenges of their goals and prepare them for possible obstacles or setbacks.

Staying aligned through purpose: caregivers can help seniors find and maintain their purpose and motivation for their goals and remind them of the reasons why they want to achieve them. Caregivers can also help seniors connect their goals to their personal values, interests, and passions and encourage them to pursue their goals with enthusiasm and joy.

Monitoring motivation and achievement: Caregivers can help seniors monitor their progress and achievement of their goals and provide them with feedback, praise, and recognition. Caregivers can also help seniors use a journal or a calendar to keep track of their activities, accomplishments, and challenges and celebrate their milestones and successes.

Finding community resources: Caregivers can help seniors access and utilize the available resources and support in their community that can help them achieve their goals. Caregivers can also help seniors find and join groups, clubs, or organizations that share their goals, interests, or hobbies and foster social connections and interactions with others.

One way to get access to a supportive network of fellow 6-minute fitness fanatics is to join the official 6-Minute Fitness Facebook group. There, you can share your progress, ask questions, and get feedback from other members. You can also participate in challenges, giveaways, and live Q&A sessions.

Another way to connect with other 6-minute fitness enthusiasts is to follow the 6-Minute Fitness Instagram account. There, you can see inspiring stories, tips, and testimonials from people who have improved their health and fitness with the 6-minute workouts. You can also comment, like, and share your own experiences.

The importance of consistency and gradual progression in exercise for seniors

Exercise is one of the best ways to maintain and improve your health and well-being as you age. However, exercise is not something that you can do sporadically or haphazardly. To reap the full benefits of exercise, you need to be consistent and gradual in your approach. Here are some reasons why consistency and gradual progression are important for exercise for seniors aged 60 and older.

Consistency means sticking to your exercise routine on a regular basis, without skipping or missing sessions. Consistency helps you build a habit of exercise, which makes it easier to overcome barriers and challenges, such as lack of time, motivation, or energy. Consistency also helps you achieve and maintain the optimal dose of exercise for your health and fitness goals, such as improving your cardiovascular, muscular, or cognitive function. Research has shown that consistent exercise can reduce the risk of chronic diseases, such as diabetes, heart disease, and dementia, and increase your life expectancy.

Gradual progression means increasing the difficulty of your exercise over time as your abilities and goals change. Gradual progression helps you avoid injury, burnout, and boredom, which can derail your exercise efforts. Gradual progression also helps you challenge yourself and improve your performance, which can boost your confidence and self-esteem. To progress gradually, start with easy exercises that suit your current ability and goals, then increase the difficulty of your exercises by performing more reps, sets, or weights, or by changing the type, intensity, or duration of your exercises.

Consistency and gradual progression are two key principles of exercise for seniors aged 60 and older. By following these principles, you can ensure that your exercise is safe, effective, and enjoyable, and that you can continue your journey toward age-defying strength and vitality.

CHAPTER 4

Longevity and Quality of Life

In the pursuit of a fulfilling and healthy life, longevity is only one part of the equation. Equally important is the quality of life experienced during those extra years.

Longevity and Quality of Life

Longevity refers to the length of a person's life, often measured in years. Advancements in healthcare and lifestyle have increased life expectancy in many parts of the world. Quality of life is a multidimensional concept encompassing physical health, mental well-being, social engagement, and overall life satisfaction. It's about living not just longer but better.

The Connection between Longevity and Quality of Life

Prolonged Independence: Living longer can be more rewarding when it's accompanied by good health and independence. Maintaining physical and mental well-being is crucial for remaining self-sufficient and active.

Fulfilling Relationships: A longer life can provide opportunities to build deeper and more meaningful relationships with family, friends, and the community. Social connections are a significant contributor to life satisfaction.

Personal Growth: Extended life allows for continuous learning and personal development. Exploring new interests and experiences can enhance mental and emotional well-being.

Legacy and Impact: A longer life can enable you to make a lasting impact on the world, leaving a meaningful legacy and contributing to the well-being of others.

Strategies for Maximizing Longevity and Quality of Life

Healthy Lifestyle Choices: Prioritize a balanced diet, regular physical activity, and stress management to maintain physical health and vitality.

Mental stimulation: Engage in activities that challenge your mind, such as learning new skills, reading, or solving puzzles, to support cognitive health.

Social Engagement: Foster and maintain meaningful social relationships to combat isolation and loneliness. Volunteer work and community involvement can contribute to a sense of purpose.

Preventive Healthcare: Regular check-ups, screenings, and vaccinations can identify and address health issues early, promoting a longer and healthier life.

Stress Reduction: Practicing relaxation techniques, meditation, or mindfulness can help reduce stress and promote emotional well-being.

Purposeful Living: Define and pursue a sense of purpose, whether it's through work, hobbies, or volunteering. Feeling a sense of meaning can positively impact life satisfaction.

Quality over quantity: Strive for a balance between living longer and living well. Quality of life should take precedence over mere longevity.

Real-life success stories of seniors who transformed their health with exercise

Exercise, as we all know, is not just good for your body but also for your mind and spirit. It can help you prevent or manage chronic diseases, improve your mood and cognition, and enhance your quality of life. Many seniors have discovered the benefits of exercise and have made remarkable changes in their health and well-being.

Here are a number of their inspiring stories

Mary Clinton, at age 72, was diagnosed with type 2 diabetes and high blood pressure. She decided to join a walking group in her neighborhood and started walking for 30 minutes every day. She also changed her diet and reduced her intake of sugar and salt. After six months, she was able to lower her blood sugar and blood pressure levels, lose 10 pounds, and feel more energetic and confident. She said walking with her friends was fun and motivating, and she enjoyed seeing nature and the people around her.

John Maxwell, at age 65, had a heart attack and underwent bypass surgery. He was depressed and afraid of having another heart attack. His doctor recommended that he join a cardiac rehabilitation program, which included supervised exercise, education, and counseling. He started with low-intensity exercises, such as cycling, swimming, and stretching, and gradually increased his intensity and duration. He also learned how to manage his stress, cope with his emotions, and adopt a healthy lifestyle. After three months, he improved his heart function, reduced his cholesterol and triglyceride levels, and regained his confidence and optimism. He said exercise helped him heal physically and mentally, and he felt like he had a second chance in life.

Linda Matthew, at age 78, had osteoporosis and arthritis. She suffered from chronic pain and stiffness in her joints and had difficulty walking and doing her daily activities. She joined a tai chi class at her local senior center, which taught her gentle and graceful movements that improved her balance, flexibility, and strength. She also practiced meditation and breathing exercises, which relaxed her mind and body. After a year, she increased her bone density, reduced her pain and inflammation, and improved her mobility and posture. She said Tai Chi made her feel calm and peaceful, and she enjoyed the social interaction and support from her classmates.

A roadmap to continuing your journey toward age-defying strength at 60+

Strength training is one of the most effective ways to maintain and improve your physical and mental health as you age. It can help you build muscle mass, increase bone density, improve balance and coordination, lower the risk of chronic diseases, and enhance your mood and self-confidence. However, strength training is not a one-size-fits-all activity. You need to consider your goals, abilities, preferences, and limitations when designing and following a strength training program. Here are some steps to help you create a roadmap for continuing your journey toward age-defying strength at 60+.

Assess your current fitness level: Before you start or modify your strength training routine, you should have a clear idea of where you are and where you want to go. You can use simple tests such as the Short Physical Performance Battery (SPPB) to measure your balance, walking speed, and ability to get out of a chair. You can also consult your doctor or a certified personal trainer to evaluate your strength, flexibility, endurance, and mobility. Based on your assessment, you can set realistic and specific goals for your strength training, such as increasing your muscle mass, improving your functional abilities, or reducing your pain.

Choose the right exercises and equipment: There are many types of strength training exercises and equipment that you can choose from, depending on your goals, preferences, and availability. Some common options include free weights, resistance bands, machines, bodyweight exercises, and functional exercises. You should aim to include exercises that target all the major muscle groups of your body, such as your chest, back, shoulders, arms, legs, and core. You should also vary your exercises and equipment periodically to avoid boredom and plateaus. You can find some examples of strength training exercises and equipment for older adults.

Determine the right intensity, frequency, and duration: The intensity, frequency, and duration of your strength training sessions will depend on your goals, fitness level, and recovery ability. As a general guideline, you should aim to perform strength training exercises at least two times per week, with at least 48 hours of rest between sessions. You should also start with a low to moderate intensity and gradually increase the resistance, repetitions, or sets as you get stronger. You should perform each exercise with proper form and technique and stop when you feel fatigue or pain. A typical strength training session for older adults should last about 20 to 30 minutes and include a warm-up and a cool-down.

Monitor your progress and adjust your program: To continue your journey toward age-defying strength, you need to track your progress and make adjustments to your program as needed. You can use various methods to monitor your progress, such as keeping a log of your exercises, weights, repetitions, and sets, measuring your body weight and body fat percentage, or repeating the SPPB or other fitness tests periodically. You can also use subjective indicators, such as how you feel, how your clothes fit, or how your daily activities have improved. Based on your progress, you can modify your program by changing the exercises, equipment, intensity, frequency, or duration to keep challenging yourself and avoid plateaus.

Seek professional guidance and support: Strength training can be a rewarding and enjoyable activity, but it can also pose some risks and challenges, especially for older adults. Therefore, it is advisable to seek professional guidance and support from your doctor, a certified personal trainer, a physical therapist, or a nutritionist. These experts can help you design a safe and effective strength training program, teach you the correct form and technique, prevent and treat injuries, and provide you with nutritional and lifestyle advice. You can also seek support from your family, friends, or other older adults who share your interest in strength training. You can join a gym, a class, a club, or an online community to find motivation, accountability, and social interaction.

Preparing for Later Life

It's crucial to plan for the later stages of life. This may involve financial preparations, such as retirement savings and long-term care insurance, as well as legal arrangements like wills and advance healthcare directives. Planning ensures that your

later years are not only comfortable but also align with your values and preferences.
Maintaining relationships and seeking purpose are all essential aspects of achieving both a longer life and a life well lived.

CHAPTER 5

Nutrition and Aging

The Role Of Nutrition in Age-Defying Strength

Nutrition plays a vital role in enhancing the benefits of strength training and promoting age-defying strength. In this chapter, we'll explore the relationship between nutrition and maintaining strength, balance, and vitality as you age.

A well-balanced diet is the foundation for supporting your body's requirements and achieving optimal results from your strength-training sweats.

Nutrient Foundations for Age-Defying Strength

Protein is essential for muscle growth and form. As we progress, our bodies may need more protein to maintain muscle mass. Include spare sources of protein in your diet, such as poultry, fish, lean meat, beans, and dairy products. Aim to spread your protein input throughout the day to support muscle recovery.

Calcium and Vitamin D: Strong bones are pivotal for overall strength and preventing fractures. Calcium and vitamin D are essential for bone health. Dairy products, fortified factory-ground milk, leafy greens, and exposure to the sun are good sources of these nutrients.

Ega-3 Adipose: Omega-3 adipose acids are known for their anti-inflammatory properties. They support common health and may reduce the threat of conditions like arthritis. Adipose fish (such as salmon and mackerel), flaxseeds, and walnuts are excellent sources.

Carbohydrates: Carbohydrates provide the energy necessary for exercise and diurnal conditioning. Choose complex carbohydrates like whole grains, fruits, and vegetables for sustained energy and proper muscle function.

Antioxidants: Antioxidants, similar to vitamins C and E, help protect your body's cells from oxidative stress. This can promote recovery and reduce inflammation after strength training. Include a variety of fruits and vegetables in your diet.

Hydration Proper: Hydration is vital for muscle function, energy, and overall health. Water is necessary for nutrient transport and waste disposal. Aim to drink an acceptable quantity of water daily, especially before and after exercise, and consider foods with high water content, such as fruits and vegetables.

Timing and balance:

The timing of your meals and snacks is pivotal to supporting your strength-training sweats. Consider these guidelines.

Pre-Workout: Consume a balanced meal or snack 1–2 hours before your strength training session. This provides the energy demanded for your drill and can enhance performance.

Post-Workout: After exercise, consume a combination of protein and carbohydrates within a couple of hours to promote muscle recovery and replenish glycogen stores.

Consistency: Constantly spacing your meals and snacks throughout the day provides your body with a steady force of nutrients to support muscle conservation and overall vitality.

Supplements

While a well-balanced diet is the preferred way to gain essential nutrients, some seniors may profit from supplements, especially if there are specific scarcities or restrictions. It's essential to consult with a healthcare provider or nutritionist before adding supplements to your routine to ensure they're safe and applicable to your requirements.

Common nutritional supplements for seniors

Multivitamins: A daily multivitamin can provide a broad variety of essential vitamins and minerals to fill implicit nutrient gaps.

Calcium and vitamin D are essential for bone health. Calcium and vitamin D supplements can help with osteoporosis and fractures.

Vitamin B12 is especially important for seniors, as B12 intake can decline with age. B12 supplements can support energy situations and neurological health.

Vitamin C is an antioxidant that supports the vulnerable system, skin health, and crack healing.

Probiotics: These supplements can help maintain digestive health and support the balance of beneficial gut bacteria. Coenzyme Q10(CoQ10) supports heart health and may ameliorate energy situations.

Magnesium is essential for muscle and whim-wham function, as well as bone health.

Iron: Some seniors may need iron supplements if they've been diagnosed with iron insufficiency, but these should be used with caution and under medical supervision.

Creating a balanced and sustainable diet is important for maintaining good health and preventing chronic diseases. A balanced diet can also help seniors feel more energetic, improve their mood, and enhance their quality of life.

Here are some tips on how to create a balanced and sustainable diet for seniors

Eat plenty of meals from specific meal groups. This will ensure that you get enough of the essential nutrients, such as protein, carbohydrates, fats, vitamins, minerals, and fiber, that your body needs.

Some examples of food groups

vegetables, fruits, whole grains, dairy, lean meats, poultry, fish, eggs, nuts, seeds, beans, and soy products.

Choose meals that might be low in added sugars, saturated fats, and sodium. These foods can increase your risk of obesity, diabetes, heart disease, and other health problems. Instead, opt for foods that are naturally sweet, such as fruits, or use natural sweeteners, such as honey or maple syrup, in moderation.

Choose foods that are high in unsaturated fats, such as olive oil, avocado, nuts, and seeds, and limit your intake of trans fats, which are found in some processed foods, such as pastries, cakes, and margarines. Reduce your salt intake by using herbs, spices, lemon juice, vinegar, or other flavorings instead of salt to season your foods.

Include protein-rich foods in every meal and snack. Protein is essential for building and maintaining muscle mass, which can decline with age. Protein also helps you feel full and satisfied, which can prevent overeating and weight gain.

Some good sources of protein

Seafood, poultry, lean meats, eggs, dairy, beans, peas, lentils, soy products, nuts, and seeds Aim for about 0.8 grams of protein per kilogram of body weight per day, or about 56 grams for a 70-kilogram (154-pound) person.

Eat more plant-based foods and less animal-based foods, such as: vegetables, fruits, whole grains, beans, nuts, and seeds, which are rich in fiber, antioxidants, phytochemicals, and other beneficial compounds that can protect your health and lower your risk of chronic diseases such as cancer, diabetes, and heart disease.

Try to eat at least five servings of fruits and vegetables per day, and choose whole grains over refined grains. Limit your intake of red meat, processed meat, and high-fat dairy, and choose lean, organic, and grass-fed options when possible.

You can also try some vegetarian or vegan meals, such as:
salads, soups, stir-fries, curries, burgers, or sandwiches that use plant-based proteins, like beans, tofu, tempeh, seitan, or nuts.

Drink plenty of water and other healthy fluids

Water is essential for hydration, digestion, absorption, circulation, and elimination. It also helps regulate your body temperature, lubricate your joints, and cushion your organs. As you age, your sense of thirst may decline, and you may lose more water through your skin and urine. This can increase your risk of dehydration, which can cause headaches, fatigue, confusion, dizziness, and other symptoms. Therefore, to prevent dehydration, drink at least eight glasses of water per day, or more if you are physically active.

You can also drink other healthy fluids, such as herbal teas, low-fat milk, soy milk, almond milk, or 100% fruit juices, but avoid sugary drinks, such as sodas, sports drinks, energy drinks, and sweetened coffee or tea, which can add extra calories and harm your teeth.
Alcohol can also dehydrate you and affect your liver, brain, and heart, so limit your intake to no more than one drink per day.

Plan your meals and snacks ahead of time.

This can help you save time, money, and effort and ensure that you have healthy foods available when you are hungry. You can use online tools, such as the USDA Food Patterns, to help you plan your meals and snacks according to your calorie and nutrient needs. You can also use cookbooks to find healthy recipes that suit your taste and budget.

Try to prepare your meals and snacks in advance and store them in the refrigerator or freezer, or you can cook in bulk and freeze the leftovers for later. You can also use a slow cooker, pressure cooker, microwave, or toaster oven to make easy and quick meals.

Enjoy your food, and eat mindfully:
Eating is not only a way to nourish your body, but also a way to enjoy your life and socialize with others. Eating should be a pleasurable and satisfying experience, not a stressful or guilt-inducing one. To

eat mindfully, pay attention to your hunger and fullness cues, and eat only when you are hungry and stop when you are full. Avoid distractions, such as TV, phone, or computer, while eating, and focus on the taste, texture, aroma, and appearance of your food. Chew your food well and eat slowly, savoring every bite. Most especially, appreciate your food and be grateful for it.

You can also make your meals more enjoyable by eating with others, such as family, friends, or neighbors, or by joining a senior center, a meal program, or a cooking club. Eating with others can also provide you with emotional support, companionship, and social interaction, which can improve your mood and well-being.

By following these tips, you can create a balanced and sustainable diet that can help you stay healthy, happy, and active for many years to come.

Remember, you are never too old to make positive changes in your eating habits and lifestyle. Start today and enjoy the benefits of a balanced and sustainable diet.

Personalized Nutrition

It's important to remember that everyone's nutritional requirements are unique. Factors like age, gender, exertion, and health conditions can impact salutary conditions. Consulting with a registered dietitian or nutritionist can help you produce a substantiated nutrition plan that aligns with your strength training intentions and supports your overall health as you age.

Incorporating sound nutrition into your life, along with regular strength training, is an important combination for age-defying strength. The relationship between nutrition and maintaining strength, balance, and vitality as you age isn't only about individual nutrients but also about the overall balance and quality of your diet. A well-balanced, nutrient-rich diet, in conjunction with regular exercise, is a holistic approach to healthy aging.

Conclusion

In the pages of "Age-Defying Strength: The 6-Minute Fitness Revolution for 60+," we've embarked on a journey toward redefining what it means to age gracefully and with vitality. Through the exploration of practical exercises and the profound impact of nutrition, we've unearthed the tools to reclaim our strength, balance, and energy.

Reducing inflammation and oxidative stress, which can damage your brain cells and impair your cognitive function. Enhancing the growth and survival of new brain cells, especially in the hippocampus, which is involved in learning and memory, improves communication and connectivity between different brain regions, which facilitates information processing and integration.

This book has not only provided a roadmap to physical well-being but has also addressed the holistic nature of aging, acknowledging the mental, emotional, and social aspects of growing older. We've recognized the role of healthcare in supporting our well-being, allowing us to navigate the complexities of the senior healthcare landscape.

In our quest for age-defying strength, we've understood that longevity is only one piece of the puzzle. The real treasure lies in the quality of those extra years, in our ability to enjoy them fully, and in the legacy we leave behind. The connection between longevity and a high quality of life is profound, and it's within our reach to make the most of both.

As we conclude our exploration, let's remember that age is just a number, and strength knows no bounds. Reclaiming vitality is not just an aspiration, it's an attainable reality. With 6 minutes a day, the power of consistency, and the wisdom shared within these pages, we can embrace the gift of aging with open arms, pursuing not just a longer life but a life of enduring strength, balance, and energy.

May the insights from this book continue to inspire, empower, and guide you in your ongoing journey of age-defying strength and a vibrant, fulfilling life.